Patchwork for Patriots

by Linda Causee

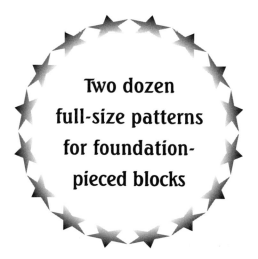

Two dozen
full-size patterns
for foundation-
pieced blocks

Introduction

Americans everywhere are looking for ways to express their patriotic spirit. Whether you are an avid quilter or a beginner to this colorful American craft, you can make a difference and show your spirit by making a patriotic patchwork project—displaying it proudly, or giving it to someone who needs comfort either here or while serving abroad.

This is a wonderful collection of foundation-pieced blocks, each with a patriotic theme. Newcomers to this technique will find complete instructions to ensure their success. You will be amazed at how easy it is to stitch small pieces of fabrics together without tedious and exact cutting of each little piece.

This collection includes two dozen full-size block patterns that can be used for wall hangings, bed quilts, sofa quilts, pot holders, pillows or wearables.

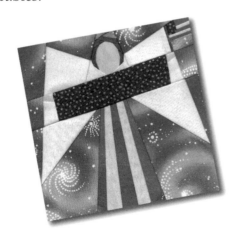

Bobbie Matela	MANAGING EDITOR
Carol Wilson Mansfield	ART DIRECTOR
Linda Causee	EDITORIAL DIRECTOR
Christina Wilson	ASSOCIATE EDITOR
Wendy Mathson	GRAPHIC DESIGNER/ EDITORIAL ASSISTANT

Blocks were foundation-pieced by
Linda Causee, Bobbie Matela
and Wendy Mathson

Thank you to the following companies who generously supplied products for our blocks:

Bernina® of America: Artista 180 sewing machine

JHB International: Buttons for cat details

Gütermann of America Inc.: 100% cotton sewing thread

For a full-color catalog including books on quilting, write to:

**American School of Needlework®
Consumer Division**
1455 Linda Vista Drive
San Marcos, CA 92069

e-mail us at: catalog@asnpub.com
visit us at: www.asnpub.com

ISBN: 1-59012-013-2   All rights reserved.   Printed in U. S. A.   3 4 5 6 7 8 9

General Directions

About the Patterns

All of the patterns in this book are full-size foundation patterns. Several of the blocks have more than one section that must be foundation-pieced individually, then sewn together. Bold lines, that are also the cutting lines, indicate these sections. A piecing diagram is included with each multi-section block showing the piecing order of the sections.

Also included with each block pattern is a shaded diagram showing the completed block. (See front and back covers for blocks in full color.) Note the finished blocks are mirror images of the original patterns, **Fig 1**.

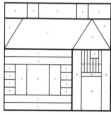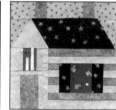

Fig 1

The Foundation Piecing Method

Foundation Material

Before you start sewing, you need to decide the type of foundation on which to piece your blocks. There are several options. Paper is a popular choice for machine piecing because it is readily available and inexpensive. Copier paper, tracing paper or newsprint work well. The paper is removed after the blocks are completely sewn.

Another alternative for foundation piecing is muslin or cotton fabric that is light-colored and lightweight for easy tracing. The fabric will add another layer that you will have to quilt through, but that is only a consideration if you are going to hand quilt. Also, if you use a fabric founda-

tion, you will be able to hand piece your blocks if that is your desire.

A third option for foundation material is Tear Away® or Fun-dation™ translucent non-woven material. Like muslin, it is light enough to see through for tracing, but like paper, it can later be easily removed before quilting.

Preparing the Foundation

Tracing the Block

Trace the block pattern carefully onto your chosen foundation material. Use a ruler and a fine-point permanent marker or fine-line mechanical pencil to make straight lines; be sure to include all numbers.

Cut 1/4" outside of the outer drawn line, **Fig 2**. Repeat for the number of blocks needed for your quilt.

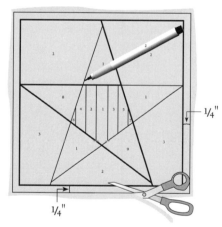

Fig 2

Transferring the Block

The block pattern can also be transferred onto foundation material, but to do this involves an additional step if you want your block to look like the shaded diagram (finished block). First, trace the block pattern onto tracing paper. Flop the paper so that the design is "backwards" and trace again onto plain paper using a transfer pen or pencil, **Fig 3**.

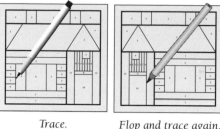

Trace.   *Flop and trace again.*

Fig 3

Then, following manufacturers' directions, iron transferred design onto foundation material. If these steps are not followed, your finished block will be a mirror image of the finished block shown, **Fig 4**.

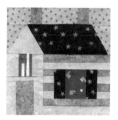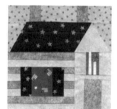

Actual block.   *Mirror image block.*

Fig 4

Fabric

We recommend using 100% cotton fabric for piecing. By using cotton rather than cotton/polyester blends, the pieces will not slip as easily and they will respond better to finger pressing.

Pre-washing fabric is not necessary, but it is advisable to test your fabric to make certain that the fabric is colorfast (don't trust manufacturers' labels). Place a 2"-wide strip (cut crosswise) of fabric into a bowl of extremely hot water; if the water changes color, the fabric is bleeding and it will be necessary to wash that fabric until all of the excess dye has washed out. Repeat for all fabrics that will be used for your quilt. Fabrics that continue to bleed after they have been washed several times should be eliminated.

3

To test for shrinkage, take each saturated strip (used previously in the colorfast test) and iron it dry with a hot iron. When the strip is completely dry, measure and compare it to your original 2" measurements. If all of your strips shrink about the same amount, then you really have no problem. When you wash your quilt, you may achieve the puckered look of an antique quilt. If you do not want this look, you will have to wash and dry all fabric before beginning so that shrinkage is no longer an issue. If any of your test strips are shrinking more than the others, these fabrics will need to be pre-washed and dried, or discarded.

Cutting the Fabric

One of biggest advantages to foundation piecing is that you do not have to cut exact pieces for every block. This is especially important for smaller blocks or blocks with many small pieces. It is much easier to handle a small section or strip of fabric than it is to handle a triangle where the finished size of the sides is 1/4".

The main consideration for using fabric pieces for a particular space is that the fabric must be at least 1/4" larger on all sides than the space it is to cover. Squares and strips are easy to figure, but triangle shapes can be a little tricky to piece. Use generous-sized fabric pieces and be careful when positioning the pieces onto the foundation. You do waste some fabric this way, but the time it saves in cutting will be worth it in the end.

Hint: *Many of the blocks contain irregularly-shaped triangles. Measure the widest point of the triangle and cut a piece of fabric 1/2" to 1" wider for piecing,* **Fig 5**.

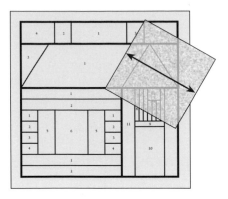

Fig 5

How to Make a Foundation-Pieced Block

1. Prepare foundations as described on the previous page in *Preparing the Foundation*. If your block has two or more sections, cut foundation apart along the bold lines, **Fig 6**.

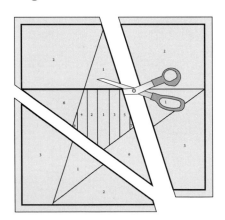

Fig 6

2. Turn foundation with unmarked side facing you and position piece 1 right side up over the space marked "1" on the foundation.

Hold foundation up to a light source to make sure that fabric overlaps at least 1/4" on all sides of space 1, **Fig 7**. Pin or use a glue stick to hold fabric in place.

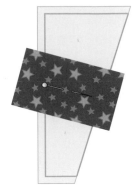

Fig 7

Hint: *Use only a small dab of a glue stick to hold fabric in place.*

3. Fold foundation back along line between space 1 and 2; trim fabric 1/4" from fold, **Fig 8**.

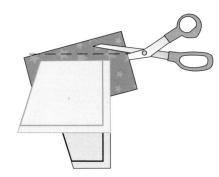

Fig 8

4. Place fabric piece 2 right sides together with piece 1; edge of fabric 2 should be even with just-trimmed edge of fabric 1, **Fig 9**.

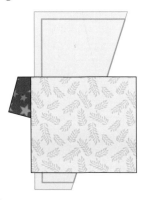

Fig 9

Double check to see if fabric piece chosen will cover space 2 completely by folding over along line between space 1 and 2, **Fig 10**.

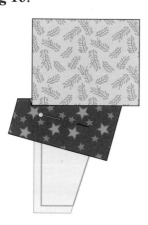

Fig 10

5. With marked side of foundation facing you, place on sewing machine, holding fabric pieces in place. Sew along line between spaces 1 and 2 using a very small stitch (18 to 20 stitches per inch), **Fig 11**. Begin and end sewing two to three stitches beyond line. You do not need to backstitch.

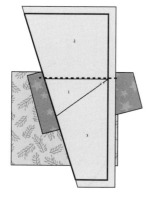

Fig 11

Hint: Sewing with a very tiny stitch will allow for easier paper removal later. If paper falls apart after stitching, your stitch length is too small and you will need to lengthen the stitch slightly.

6. Turn foundation over. Open piece 2 and finger press seam, **Fig 12**. Use a pin or dab of glue stick to hold piece in place if necessary.

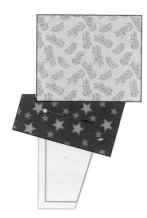

Fig 12

7. Turn foundation with marked side of foundation facing you; fold foundation forward along line between spaces 1 and 3 and trim about $1/8"$ to $1/4"$ from fold, **Fig 13**.

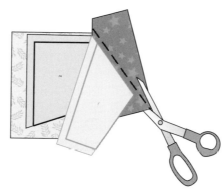

Fig 13

Hint: If using a paper foundation, carefully pull paper away from stitching for easier trimming. If using a fabric foundation, fold it forward as far as it will go and trim.

8. Place fabric 3 right side down, even with just-trimmed edge, **Fig 14**.

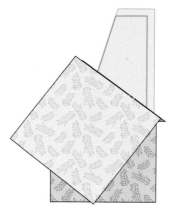

Fig 14

9. Turn foundation to marked side and sew along line between spaces 1 and 3; begin and end sewing two to three stitches beyond line, **Fig 15**.

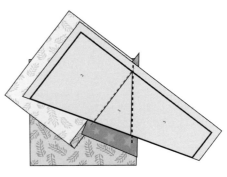

Fig 15

10. Turn foundation over, open piece 3 and finger press seam, **Fig 16**. Glue or pin in place.

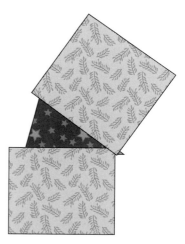

Fig 16

11. Trim 1/4" from outside drawn line of foundation, **Fig 17**. Note the cut edge of the foundation is 1/4" from outside edge of block.

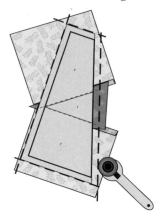

Fig 17

12. Continue trimming and sewing pieces in numerical order in remaining sections, **Fig 18**. Make sure pieces along the outer edge are large enough to allow for the 1/4" seam allowance.

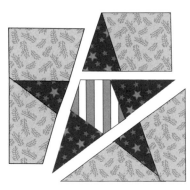

Fig 18

13. Press section, then trim fabric 1/4" from outside line of foundation block to complete block (or section).

Hint: *Do not remove paper yet. It is better to remove paper after blocks have been sewn together. Since grain line wasn't considered in piecing, outer edges may be on the bias and, therefore, stretchy. Keeping paper in place until after sewing will prevent the blocks from becoming distorted.*

Staystitching along outer edge of block, Fig 19, will also help keep fabric from stretching out of shape. If stay stitching, you may remove paper prior to sewing blocks together.

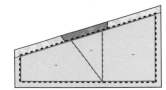

Fig 19

14. Some of the blocks have two or more sections. To sew together, place sections right sides together; push a pin through corner of top section going through to corner of bottom section, **Fig 20**.

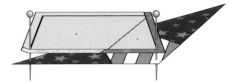

Fig 20

15. Check to be sure pin goes through both corners and is perpendicular (going straight up) to block. If not, pin again until corners match. Repeat at opposite corner to match seams. Once pieces are lined up correctly, sew along edge of foundation using a regular stitch length, **Fig 21**.

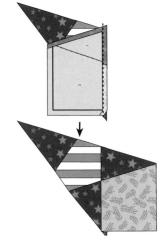

Fig 21

Hint: *If desired, baste sections together by hand or machine. Check sections again; if everything matches up, sew together with regular stitches. Basting*

takes a little time, but the extra effort will be worth it in the end.

16. Sew all sections together in same manner to complete block, **Fig 22**, referring to piecing diagram.

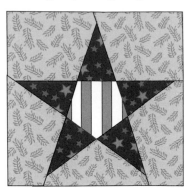

Fig 22

Highlights and Hints for Foundation Piecing

- Begin and end sewing at least two to three stitches beyond line you are sewing on, **Fig 23**.

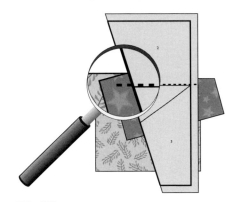

Fig 23

- Some of the blocks have very tiny pieces, so don't worry if your stitching goes through a whole space and into another space, **Fig 24**; it will not interfere with adding subsequent pieces.

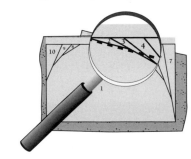

Fig 24

- Use a short stitch, around 20 stitches per inch.
- Trim seam allowances 1/8" to 1/4" (or smaller if necessary).
- Finger press or press with an iron after every seam. The little wooden "irons" found in quilt shops or catalogs work great.
- When sewing spaces with points, it is easier to start from the wide end and sew towards the point, **Fig 25.**

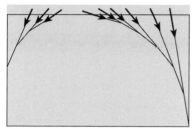

Fig 25

- Don't worry too much about grainline. Sewing to a foundation stabilizes the fabric and will prevent it from getting out of shape.
- Directional prints are not recommended unless they are used only once in a block or placed where they can be used easily in a consistent manner, **Fig 26**.

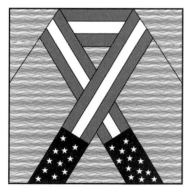

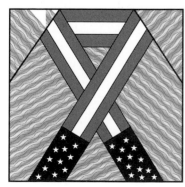

Fig 26

Basic Embroidery Stitches

Facial features in the "Freedom Feline" block were embroidered with a stem stitch, as demonstrated below.

Stem Stitch

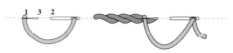

Bring needle up at 1. Hold thread down with thumb of your non-stitching hand. Reinsert needle at 2 and bring up at 3, about halfway between 1 and 2. Pull thread through and continue in this manner with thread held below stitching. Work in straight or curved lines.

Satin stitch embroidery can be used to fill in cat's eyes and nose, instead of using buttons as in our sample block.

Satin Stitch

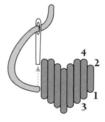

Come up at 1 and down at 2. Continue with straight stitches very close together to fill desired pattern.

Finishing Your Quilt

Making the Quilt Top

Make the number of blocks needed for desired quilt size. All blocks finish 7" square. Lay out blocks in a pleasing arrangement. Sew quilt blocks together in rows; press seams for rows in alternate directions. Sew rows together, matching seams.

To add borders, measure quilt top lengthwise; cut two border strips to that length and sew to sides of quilt. Measure quilt top crosswise, including borders just added; cut two border strips to that length. Sew to top and bottom edges of quilt top. Repeat for any additional borders. Remove paper foundations at this time.

Layering the Quilt

There are many types of batting on the market. Use batting that is suitable for the use of your quilt. If making a wallhanging, choose a thin cotton or polyester batting. If making a bed quilt, you may want a low-loft polyester batting for a little more thickness. Check the label to see the quilting requirements and follow those guidelines.

Use 100% cotton fabric for the backing of your quilt. For quilts wider than the 40"- to 44"-wide fabric, you will have to piece your backing unless you use the 90"- to 106"- wide fabrics that are currently available.

Cut backing and batting about 1" to 2" larger on all sides than the quilt top. Place backing wrong side up, then smooth out batting on top. Center quilt top right side up on batting.

Baste layers together using one of the following techniques:

Fusible Iron-on Batting – The new Fusible Batting™ by June Tailor is a wonderful new way to hold the quilt layers together without using other time-consuming methods of basting.

Thread basting – Baste with long stitches, starting in center and sewing toward edges in a number of diagonal lines.

Safety pin basting – Pin through all layers at once, starting from center and working toward edges. Place pins no more than 4" apart, thinking of your quilt plan as you work to make certain pins avoid prospective quilting lines.

Quilt gun basting – Use the handy trigger tool (found in quilt and fabric stores) that pushes nylon tags through all layers of the quilt. Start in center and work randomly toward outside edges. Place tags about 4" apart. You can sew right over the tags and then easily remove them by cutting off with a pair of scissors.

Spray or heat set basting – Use one of the spray adhesives currently on the market, following manufacturer's directions.

Quilting

If you have never used a sewing machine for quilting, you might want to read more about the technique. *Learn to Machine Quilt in Just One Weekend* (ASN #4186), by Marti Michell, is an excellent introduction to machine quilting. This book is available at your local quilt or fabric store, or write the publisher for a list of sources.

You do not need a special machine for quilting. Just make sure your machine is oiled and in good working condition. An even-feed foot is a good investment if you are going to machine quilt, since it is designed to feed the top and bottom layers of the quilt through the machine evenly.

Use fine transparent nylon thread in the top and regular sewing thread in the bobbin.

To **quilt in-the-ditch** of a seam (this is actually stitching in the space between two pieces of fabric that have been sewn together), use your fingers to pull blocks or pieces apart slightly and machine stitch right between the two pieces. Try to keep stitching to the side of the seam that does not have the bulk of the seam allowance under it. When you have finished stitching, the quilting will be practically hidden in the seam.

Free form machine quilting is done with a darning foot and the feed dogs down on your sewing machine. It can be used to quilt around a design or to quilt a motif. Free form machine quilting takes practice to master because you are controlling the movement of the quilt under the needle, rather than the machine moving the quilt. With free form machine quilting, you can quilt in any direction: up and down, side to side and even in circles, without pivoting the quilt around the needle.

Attaching the Binding

Trim backing and batting even with quilt top. For side edges, measure the quilt top lengthwise; cut two 2½"-wide strips that length. Fold strips in half lengthwise wrong sides together. Place one strip along one side of the quilt; sew with a ¼" seam allowance, **Fig 27**.

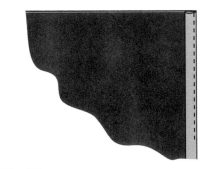

Fig 27

Turn binding to back and slipstitch to backing, covering previous stitching line, **Fig 28**. Repeat on other side.

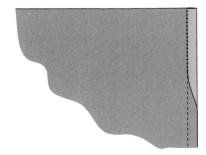

Fig 28

For top and bottom edges, measure quilt crosswise and cut two 2½"-wide strips that length, adding ½" to each end. Fold strips in half lengthwise with wrong sides together. Place one strip along top edge with ½" extending beyond each side; sew with a ¼" seam allowance, **Fig 29**.

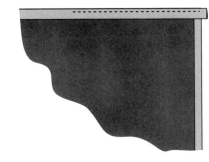

Fig 29

Turn binding to back and tuck the extra ½" under at each end; slipstitch to backing fabric. Repeat at bottom edge.

The Finishing Touch

After your quilt is finished, always sign and date it. A label can be cross stitched, embroidered or even written with a permanent marking pen. To make decorative labels in a hurry, *Iron-on Transfers for Quilt Labels* (ASN #4188) and *Foundation-Pieced Quilt Labels* (ASN #4196), provide many patterns for fun and unique quilt labels. Hand stitch to back of quilt.

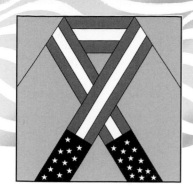

Remembrance Ribbon

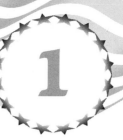

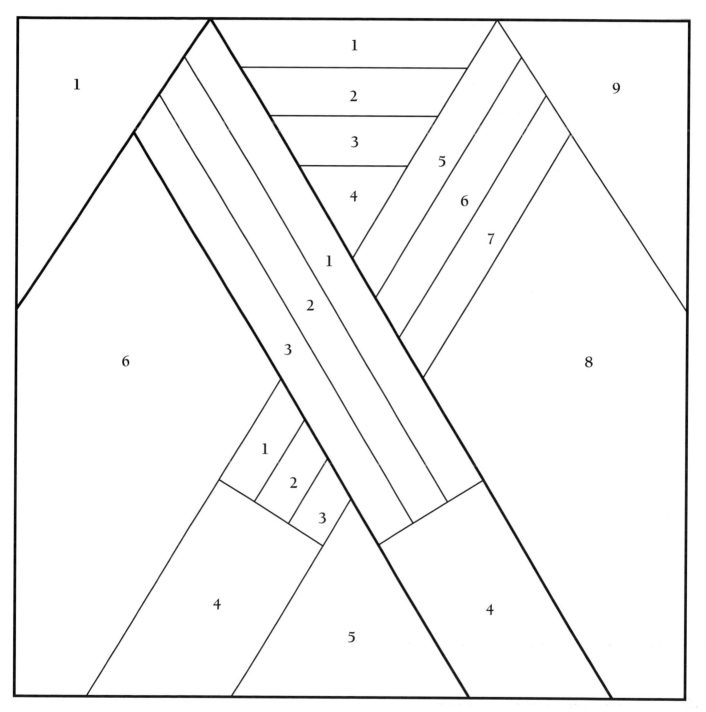

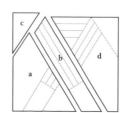

Overall Uncle Sam

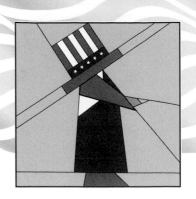

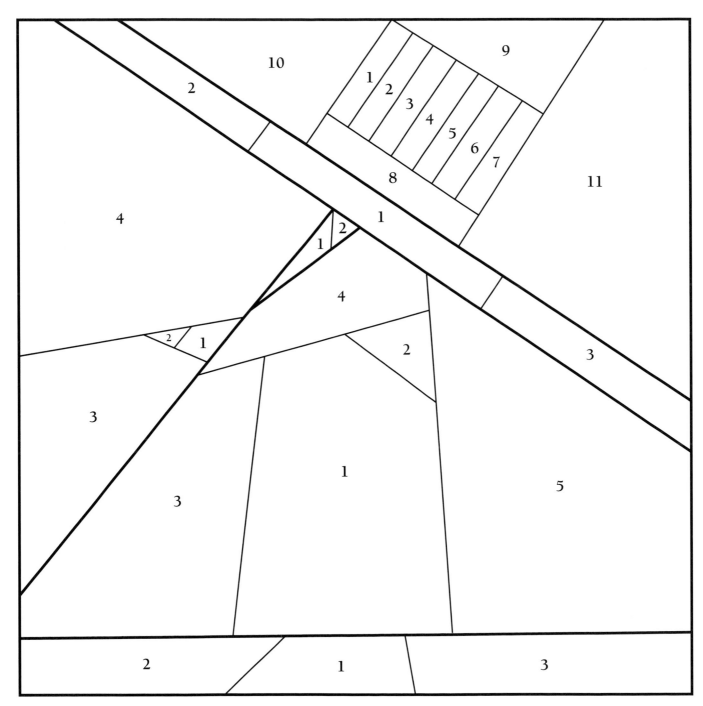

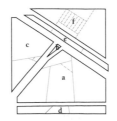

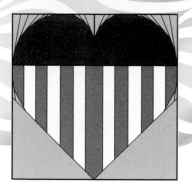

Stars & Stripes Heart

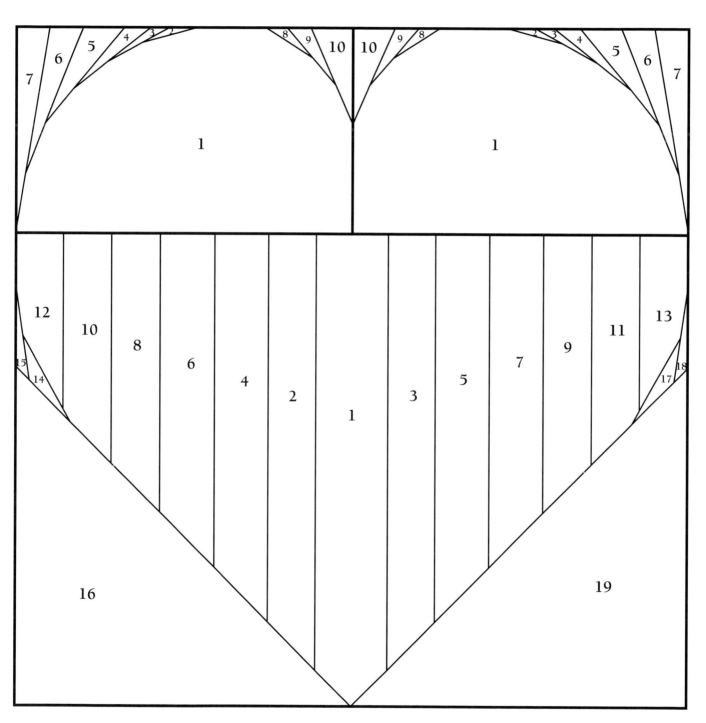

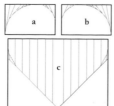

Sunbonnet Betsy Ross

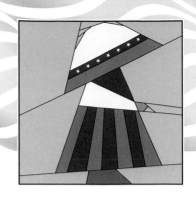

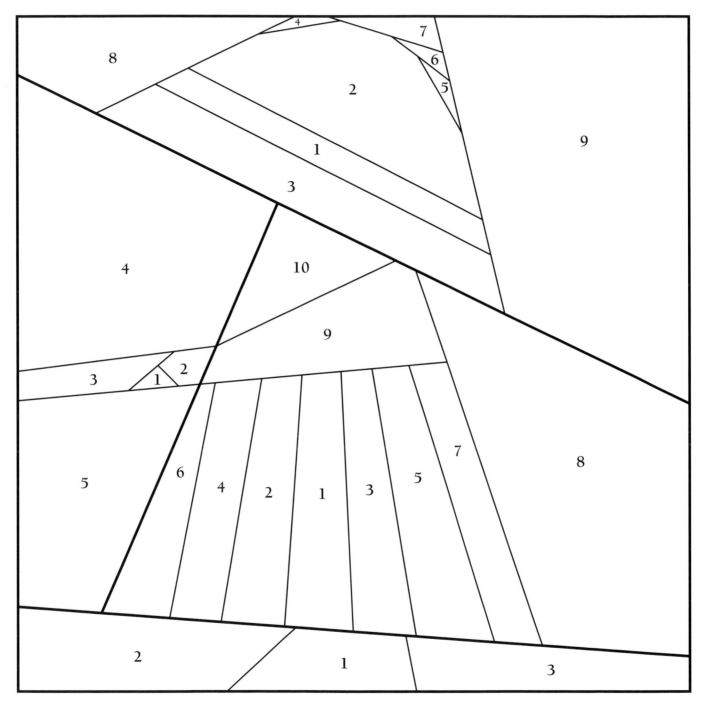

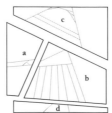

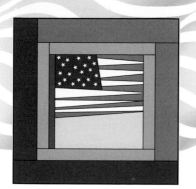

Old Glory

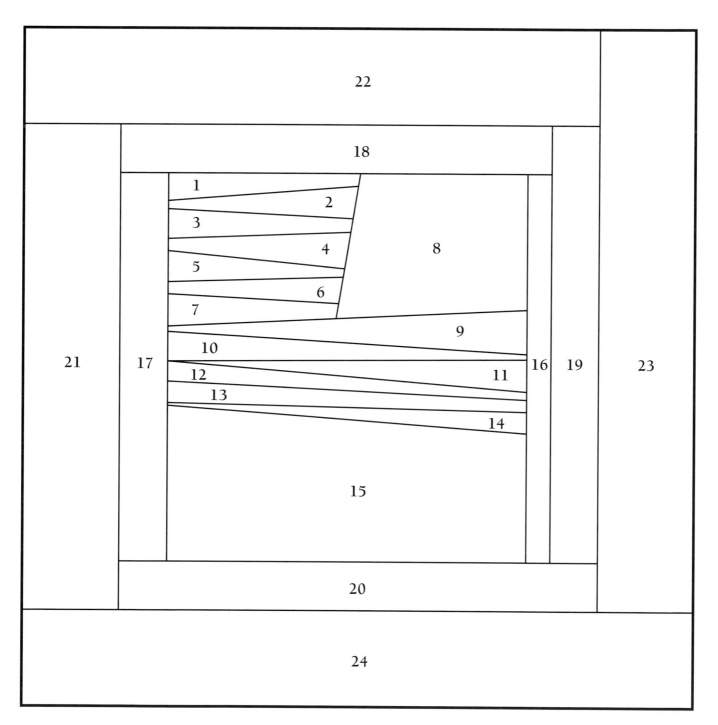

Angel of Liberty

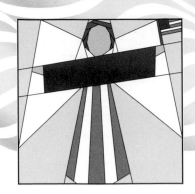

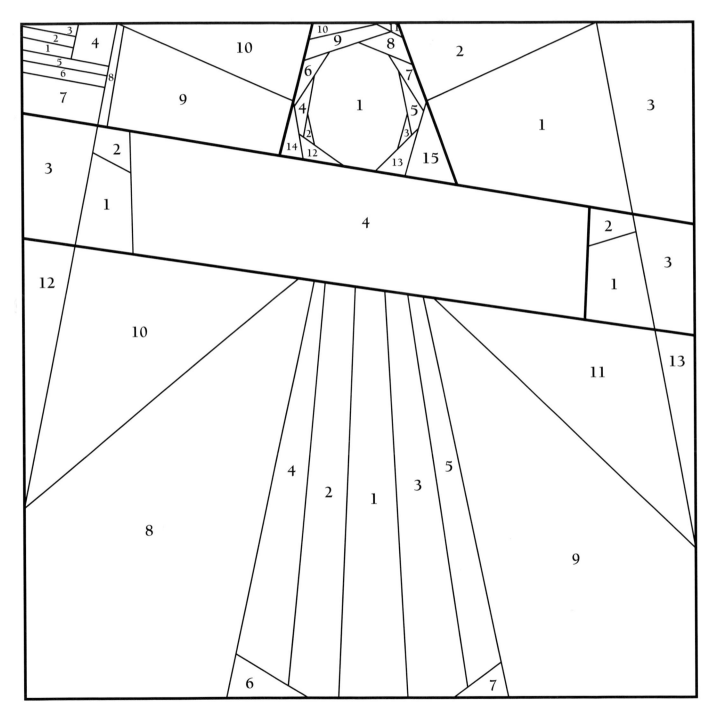

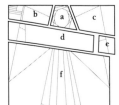

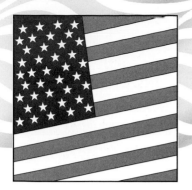

Flag Unfurled

6

4

2

1

3

5

7

8

9

10

11

12

13

14

The Big Apple

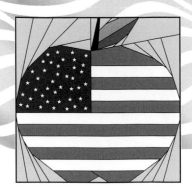

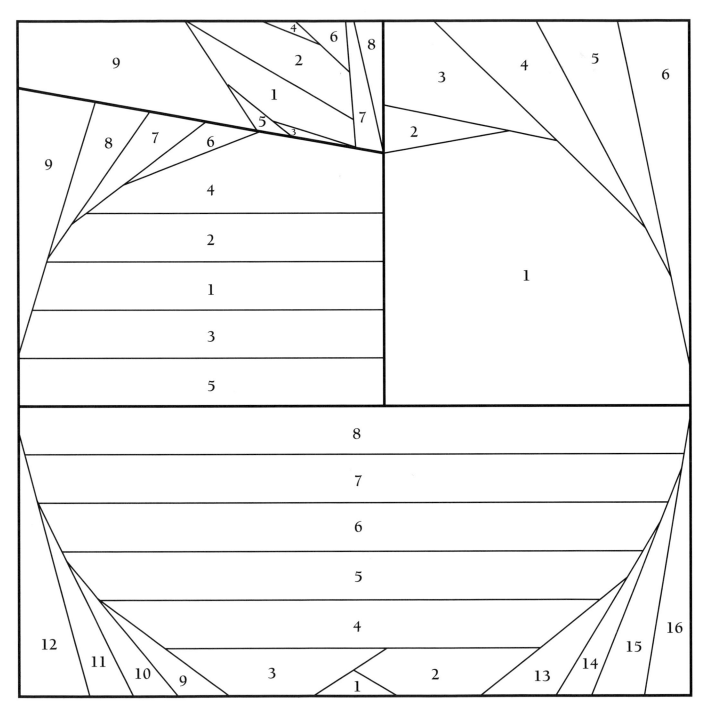

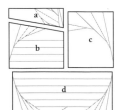

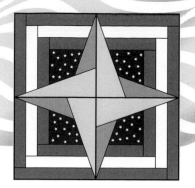

Golden Star

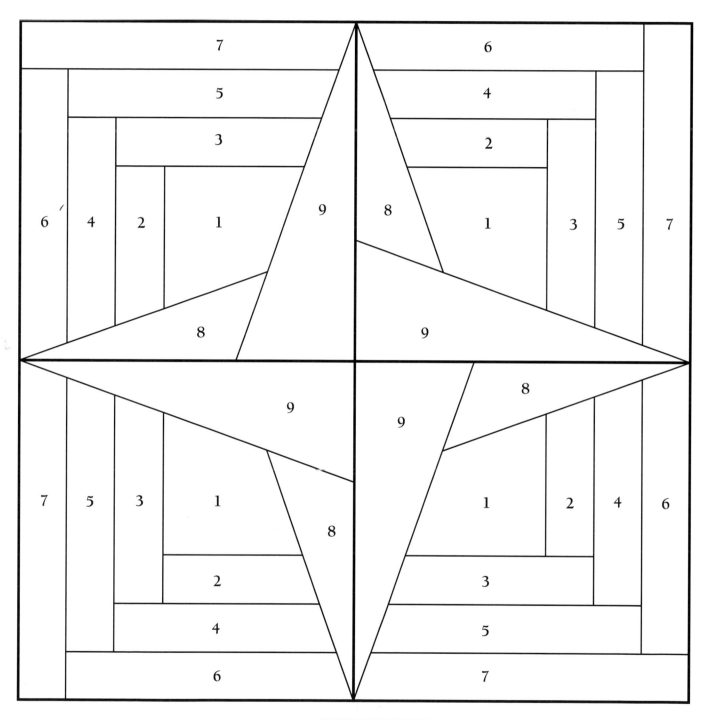

7					6
5				4	
3			2		

6 4 2 1 9 8 1 3 5 7

8 9

9 8

9 9

8

7 5 3 1 1 2 4 6

8

2 3

4 5

6 7

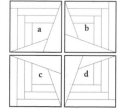

Proud Pinwheel

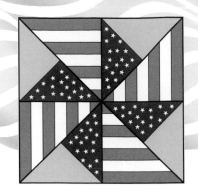

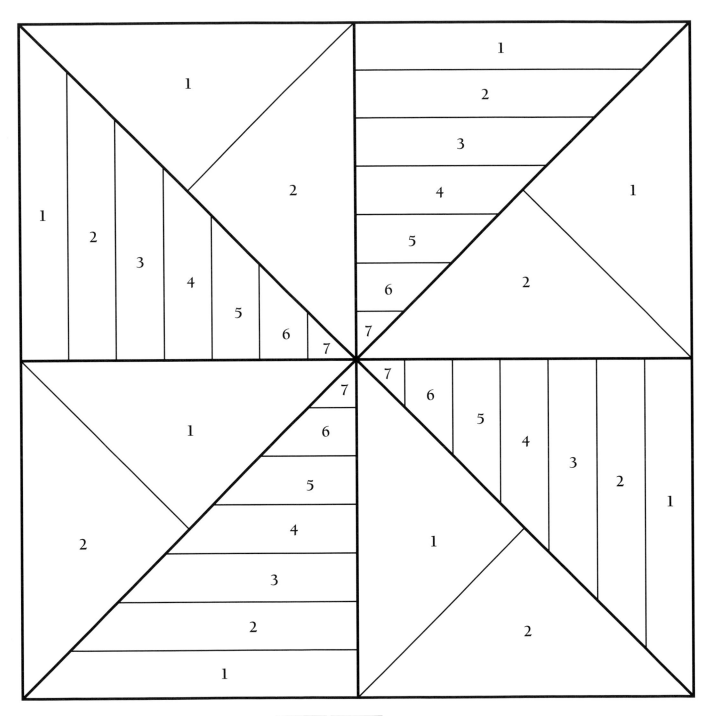

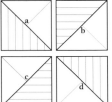

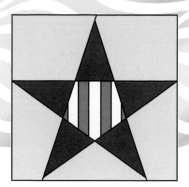

Spirit Star

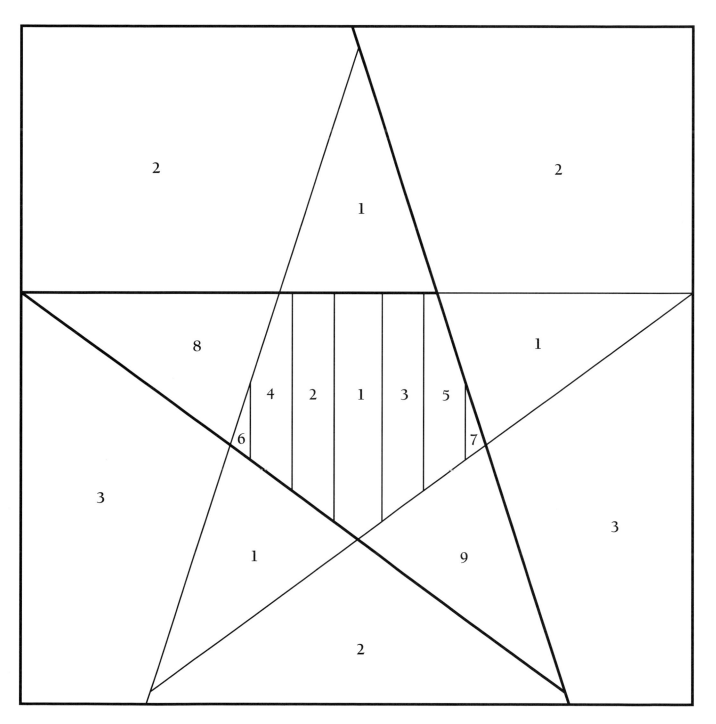

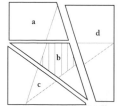

Independence
Log Cabin

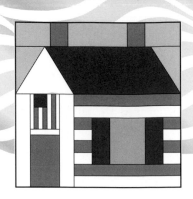

| 4 | 2 | 1 | 3 | 5 |

| 3 | 1 | 4 |
| | | 2 |

| 1 |
| 2 |

1	5	6	5	1
2				2
3				3
4				4

| 4 |
| 8 | 7 | 5 | 2 | 1 | 3 | 6 |
| 11 | 9 | 12 |
| 10 |

| 1 |
| 2 |

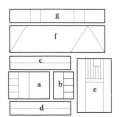

g

f

c

a   b   e

d

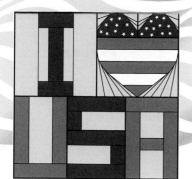

I ♥ USA

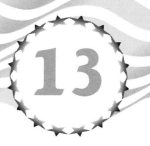

Heart (left): 4 3 2 1 7 6 5

Heart (right): 7 6 5 1 4 3 2

Large heart block:
1
2
3
4
10 9 8 7 6 5 11 12 13 14 15

Right upper block:
4
6 2 1 3 7
5

Lower left block:
6
2
4 1 5
3

Center lower block:
3
1 2
3
2 1
4

Lower right block:
2 1 3
4

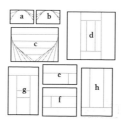

a b
c
d
g
e
f
h

Freedom Feline

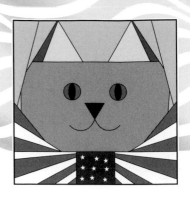

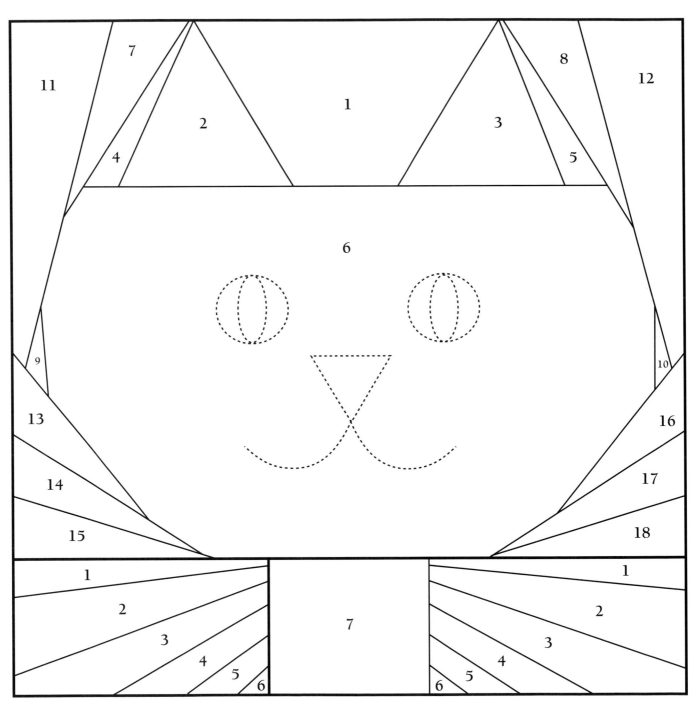

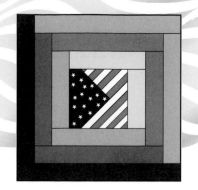
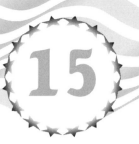
24

20

16

5 6 7

4

3

2

1

23 19 15 8 17 21 25

9

10

11

12

13

14

18

22

26

Liberty Bell

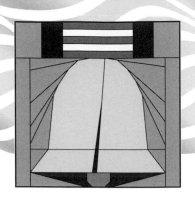

Top section:

8	6		7	9
		4		
		2		
		1		
		3		
		5		

Main section:

13   8

12   7

11   6

1   3   2   1

10   5

9   4

1

5   4

3   1   2

6   4   1   5   7

2   3

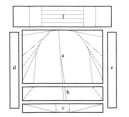

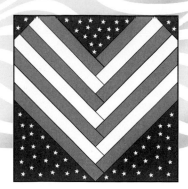

Show-Your-Stripes Heart

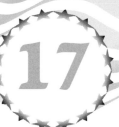

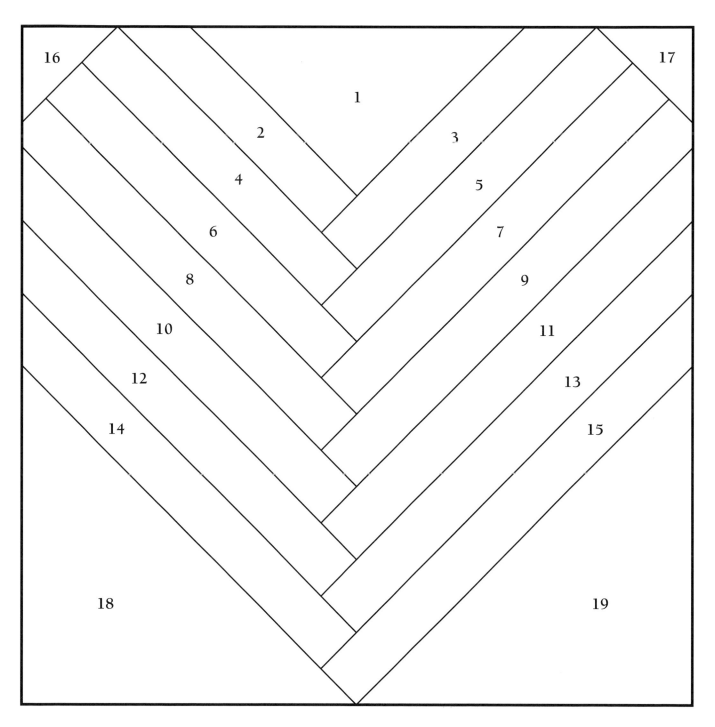

Star Spangled USA

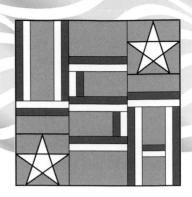

Block 1 (left):

2		2
1	1	1
3	2	3	3
1		

| 11 |
| 10 |
| 9 |

7	5	3		6	8
		1		
		2		
		4		

Block 2 (center):

| 6 |
| 5 |
| 4 |

| 1 | 2 | 3 |

| 5 |
| 4 |

| 3 | 2 | 1 |

| 6 |
| 7 |

| 8 |

Block 3 (right):

| 4 | 2 | 1 | 3 | 5 |

| 6 |
| 7 |
| 8 |

| 2 | | 2 |
| 2 |
| 1 | 1 |
| 1 |
| 2 | 2 | 2 | 3 |
| 1 |

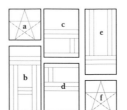

a c e
b d f

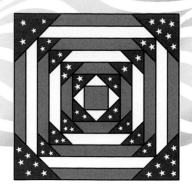

American Pineapple

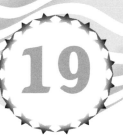

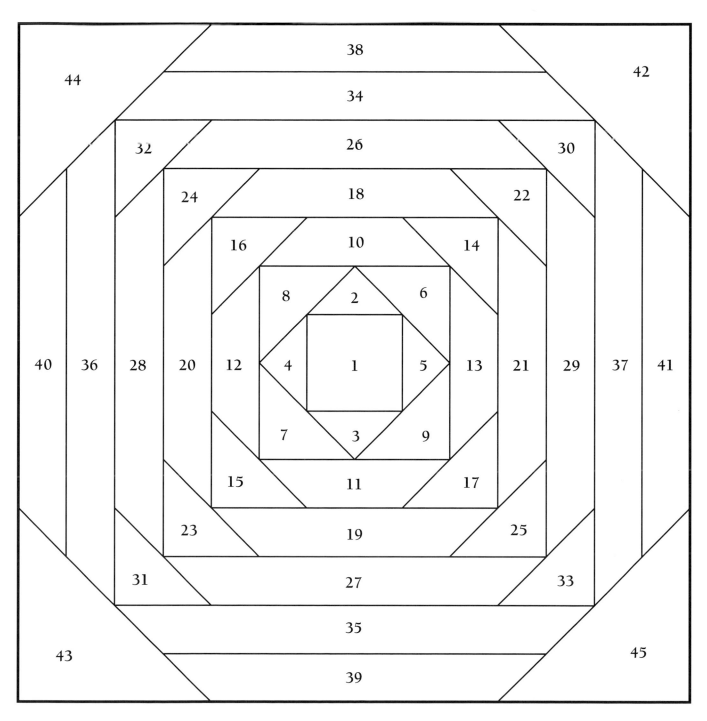

Anchors Aweigh!

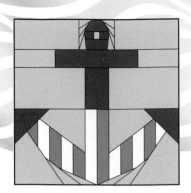

12	13

Top boat section:
- 10, 11
- 8, 9
- 2, 1, 3
- 6, 7
- 4, 5

2	1	3

2	1	3

Left section:
- 11
- 5
- 4
- 6
- 3
- 2
- 1
- 7
- 10
- 9
- 8

Right section:
- 6
- 11
- 5
- 7
- 4
- 3
- 2
- 1
- 10
- 8
- 9

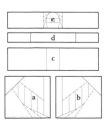

e

d

c

a   b

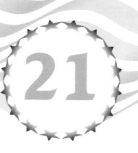
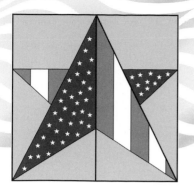

Patriot's Star

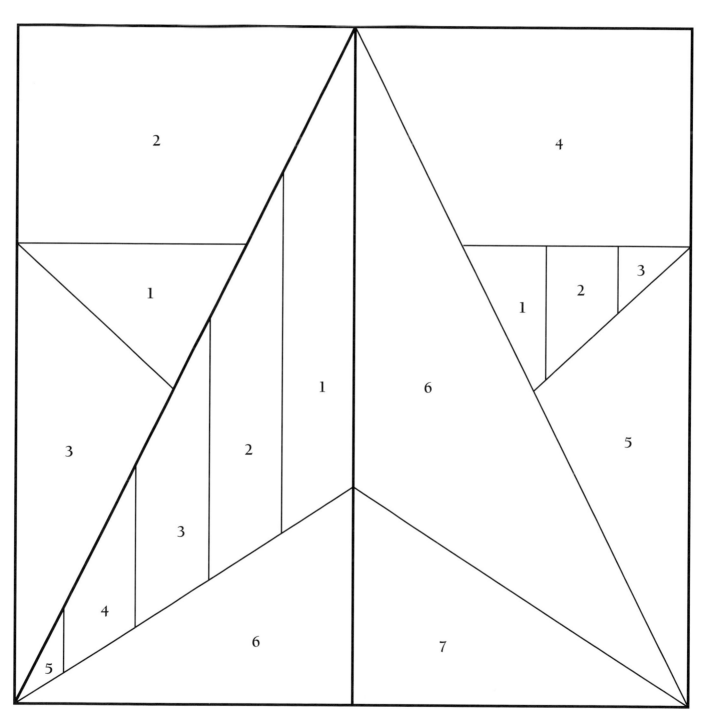

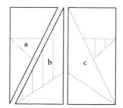

Ohio Star Flag

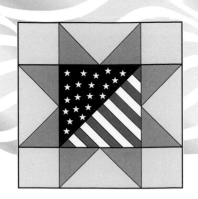

```
┌──────────┬──────────────────┬──────────┐
│          │        1         │          │
│    4     │                  │    5     │
│          │   2          3   │          │
├──────────┼──────────────────┼──────────┤
│          │ 12               │    3     │
│    3     │  10              │          │
│          │   8              │          │
│          │    6          14 │          │
│    1     │     4            │    1     │
│          │      2           │          │
│          │       1          │          │
│    2     │        3         │    2     │
│          │         5        │          │
│          │          7       │          │
│          │           9      │          │
│          │          11      │          │
│          │            13    │          │
├──────────┼──────────────────┼──────────┤
│          │   2          3   │          │
│    4     │                  │    5     │
│          │        1         │          │
└──────────┴──────────────────┴──────────┘
```

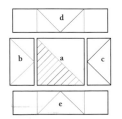

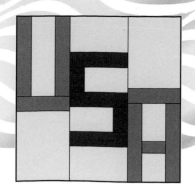

USA Pride

7	4	2 1 3
	3	
	1 2	
6	3	4
2	2 1	5
4 1 5	4	
3	5	

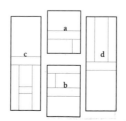

Patriotic Pinwheel

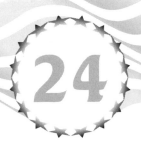

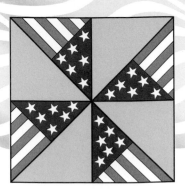

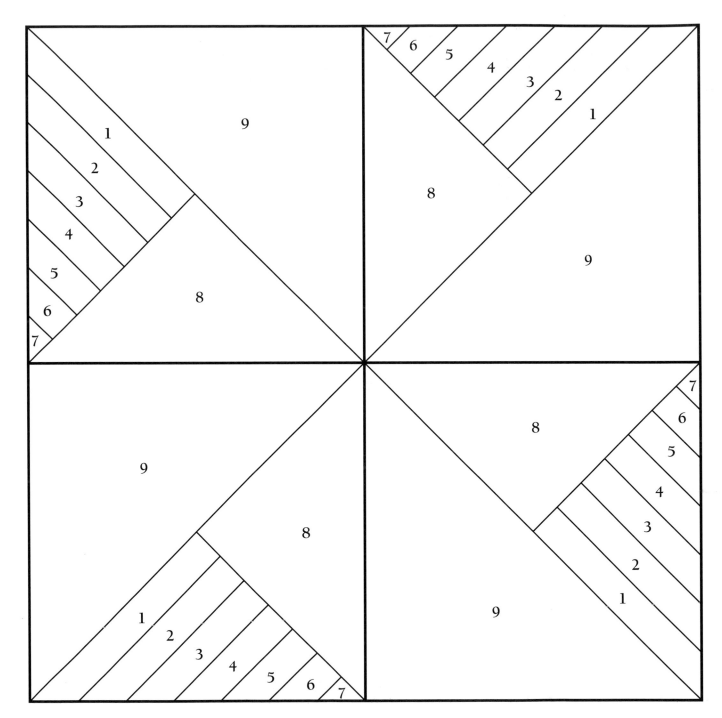